The Most Natural and Effective Ways to Quit Smoking

Easy-to-Do Steps to End the Cigarette Habit Forever

By: Allan Doe

9781681275222

D0274510

PUBLISHERS NOTES

Disclaimer – Speedy Publishing LLC

This book was originally printed before 2014. This is an adapted reprint by Speedy Publishing LLC with newly updated content designed to help readers with much more accurate and timely information and data.

Speedy Publishing LLC

40 E Main Street, Newark, Delaware, 19711

Contact Us: 1-888-248-4521

Website: http://www.speedypublishing.co

REPRINTED Paperback Edition: 9781681275222:

Manufactured in the United States of America

DEDICATION

This book is dedicated to my cousin, Phoebe. Your fight against nicotine has been nothing short of inspiring. Thank you for allowing me to share it to the rest of the world.

TABLE OF CONTENTS

Chapter 1- End the Cigarette Habit Today

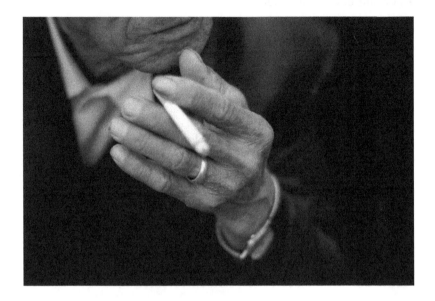

It may not necessarily be easy to do but there has been a multitude of people who have already made the decision to quit smoking and have successfully done so. When you know what to expect you will position yourself for to be successful in your attempt to quit. In addition to feeling better you will reap many other benefits from your decision to stop smoking.

Personal Health

The main reason people usually make the decision to quit smoking is centered on health issues. It is a known fact that smoking can cause lung cancer but it can do many other things as well to your health

• Various other cancers in addition to lung cancer

• Emphysema and chronic bronchitis,

• Heart condition increasing risk for heart attack

• Peripheral vascular disease,

• Increased risk for stroke

• Premature aging of the skin, bad breath, bad smelling clothes and hair and yellowing of fingernails.

• Increased risk during pregnancy including miscarriages and lower birth-weight babies

No matter how long you have smoked, when you quit smoking you will benefit from doing so. If you stop smoking before age 35 you can actually prevent 90% of the health risk associated with smoking. To quit smoking later in life will still provide benefits and reduce the risk of diseases associated with smoking.

Cost

In addition to improving your health and lower your risk for certain diseases another reason to quit smoking is the cost to smoke. Smoking is an expensive habit and most people that smoke could use the money they spend for smoking for other things needed in their life. The annual cost for the average smoker is estimated to be approximately 3,391 dollars.

Calculate quickly how much you spend in a year smoking: consider how much you spend in a day and multiply it by 365. To look at how much you have already spent in your lifetime multiply the amount you spend per year by the number of years you have been smoking. Surprised at the amount of money you might say you have simply burnt up? Change that today by making a decision to quit smoking now.

Still haven't decided to quit smoking? Let's look at this another way, take the amount you spend per year smoking and multiple it by 10 assuming you continue to smoke for the next 10 years. Wow, that is a lot of money! Just think that is money you have not spent yet, so if you decide to quit smoking today, just what could you do with that money?

This has only included the cost of the cigarettes not the additional cost of insurance and healthcare due to the effects of continuing to smoke.

Alternatives to Smoking

Yes, there are truly people who just can't imagine what they could possibly do in certain situations if they did not smoke. Perhaps you have even thought this about yourself. Do you find you must smoke when you are sad, happy, stressed, troubled, or tired? So if you quit smoking, what will you do?

First let's take a look at what that cigarette is doing for you in these types of situations.

If you are happy and want to celebrate and you have that cigarette in your hand and now you start to reach over to give someone a celebration hug. What is in the way? You got it the cigarette. Perhaps you often will stop and lay aside your cigarette so you can celebrate with a hug for someone. Now tell me, how that cigarette helped you celebrate. Oh, I see by getting in the way.

Let's move on your sad, perhaps you just found out you didn't get that big raise at work. So the first thing you reach for is a cigarette. Oh now this is really good. You are sad because you are not going to get more money in your paycheck so what is you answer get a cigarette put fire to the end of it and burn it up. How much did that cigarette cost you and how much is that next doctor bill going to be due to the effects on your body of smoking. So now you are getting the raise and you just spent or better said burnt up some of your existing money. That should really make you feel better, Right?

Nothing can put stress on people like having health problems and the worry it can bring. Your doctor just called to tell you he ordered another chest x-ray because "something" showed up on the first one Just like a magnet your hand reaches over for another cigarette. Why, because you are stressed due to worry about what that "something" was that just showed up on the last x-ray. What is that cigarette going to do for whatever the "something" is? Get the point you just added a problem on top of a problem and you thought that was helping.

You teenager didn't get home on time last night and you were worried. You've got trouble on your hands and the first thing you want in your hands with that trouble is a cigarette. You are going to talk with your teenager about how they need to follow the rules and be home on time so others do not worry and it is for their own good. All the stuff parents say with a cigarette in your hand which you know is not good for you. Oh I get it, Son do as I say not as I do.

You've worked hard all day and finally you are home relaxed in your favorite chair and you reach over for a cigarette to help you rest. And rest you do, cigarette in hand and just about the time you doze off the smoke alarm goes off. Forget about being tired now you have to put a fire out that started in the chair. Oops was it from that cigarette you wanted to help relax with.

The thing to do is quit smoking today.

CHAPTER 2- WHERE SHOULD YOU START?

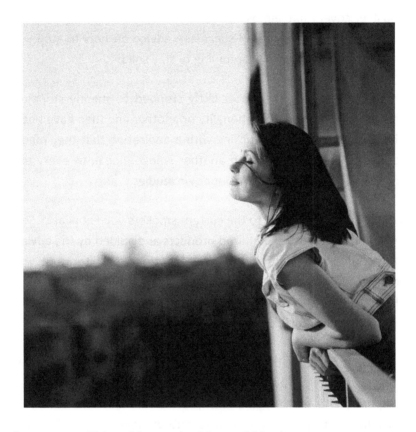

I suppose utilizing this standard it would be best not to trust me. But prior to jumping ship there's one additional crucial group of individuals that you might discover that will back me up and who are already rather credible to you. It's the individuals in your family unit and your acquaintances in your real life that have successfully stopped smoking and been off any nicotine products for at the least one year or more.

Discover how the individuals you know who are long-run ex-smokers really quit smoking. By long-run I mean individuals who are presently off all nicotine for at the least a year or more. You will probably discover that few if any of them know who I am.

Self-Diagnosis, Healing and Recovery

You'll determine that a lot of them had former quits and regressed, utilizing all types of techniques that are supported by pros and perhaps even a couple of them had pro help with old attempts. You'll discover that almost all of them didn't abide by what is believed to be the standard suggested advice on how to stop yet they did stop and are still continuing to stay solid.

You'll discover that they most likely stopped by merely stopping smoking one day for one rationality or another and then have been able to remain there by sticking with a dedication that they made to themselves to not pick up another smoke. Speak to every ex-smoker you'll understand. Do your own studies.

While you're at it, speak to the current smokers you know also. See how many of them have utilized products and abided by the advice of the pros. Bear in mind, a lot of professional literature will counsel individuals to utilize pharmacologic aids like nicotine alternate products. Attempt to see how many long-run successful quitters in your real life encounters really abided by this advice.

A different piece of advice composed in most literature created by smoking cessation authorities is something to the effect that temporary errs are usual and that you shouldn't let a err send you back to smoking. Individuals who author advice like this don't comprehend addiction. An individual needs to comprehend that taking just one puff is likely going to kill your attempts at quitting.

If you listen to, "don't let a slip make you return to smoking," you may sadly, find out from experience that you have little control of the matter once you take that puff.

Our advice, if to successfully stop smoking, is to merely quit smoking. Our advice for keeping off cigarettes is merely to stick with a dedication to never pick up another cigarette. So talk to long-run ex-smokers and discover how they stopped and hear how they've managed to keep off them.

Pretty soon you'll see it isn't a matter of matching all of the world pros against me. It gets to be a matter of matching every long-run ex-smoker you know who's successfully stopped against the world's pros. Do the studies and then I'll simply become a different voice in the crowd of real individuals who have demonstrated to you that the way to stop smoking and to stay smoke free is to - never pick up another smoke and quit today...put them down!

Which Method Should You Choose?

The vast array of methods to choose from to quit smoking can actually make the task of choosing a method practically as difficult as stopping to smoke. With so much information available regarding different methods many experience information overload and never select a quit smoking method at all but continue to smoke. Let's look at some simple but successful methods to quit smoking.

First you should plan your strategy to quit smoking. A simple direct plan should be developed no matter which quit smoking method you select. A suggestion is the KISS approach which is keeping it simple stupid.

Ask yourself the question why or when do I smoke? If you find yourself smoking in certain circumstances or perhaps when you are in certain moods, stop and take a second look, deal with the situation, and don't reach for those cigarettes. Although smoking is an addiction, perhaps you continue to smoke due to stress or other feelings. It is necessary to deal with these situations before attempting to stop smoking.

Self-Diagnosis, Healing and Recovery
If you are not careful, you can put together a very difficult plan that will leave you very little room for success.

Finding a substitution for your smoking habit can prove beneficial. Some examples of substitute activities include:

• Find something you enjoy to do, such as art or sports.

• Incorporate your new hobby into your daily schedule

Include in your quit smoking plan any substitutions you have identified as well as incorporating these substitutions into your daily schedule. Conquering your urge to smoke is a necessary to be successful. Keeping it simple depends upon how difficult you make it to be. Learn the most effective quit smoking method.

It's Your Choice to Make

Each of our lives is actually the result of our choices. Yes we choose most of the things in life. We choose what we are going to wear, what we are going to eat, who are life partner will be, what are career will be, and yes it is a choice that is made to smoke or quit smoking.

Yes you choose to smoke or not to smoke. Cigarettes do not find their own way into your mouth. You have made the choice to place each cigarette you have ever smoked into your mouth. You even made the choice to buy the cigarettes at the store.

From the time you first have an urge for a cigarette you make choices that lead to the eventual smoking of that cigarette. You take your money to the store and purchase a pack of cigarettes that was your choice. You open the pack of cigarettes and remove one, light it, and smoke it that was your choice. How many times

Allison McPhee

have you made that special trip to the store just to purchase cigarettes? Now wasn't that a lot of work for a pack of cigarettes.

You want a cigarette and you are out. You could choose to not go buy that new pack today rather than going to all that work just to get a pack of cigarettes. Why not decide or rather choose to quit smoking right then. What better time could there be?

Our lives really are the after effect of all the choices we make on a daily basis. And practically all of the choices we make with complete freedom to choose what we want.

These choices can bring us prosperity or poverty; make us sad or happy, satisfied or dissatisfied and a smoker or non-smoker.

Your choice to not smoke could be influenced by the desire to have good health, improve your financial situation, not smell like smoke, or have more energy. When you decide to quit smoking you need to choose things to replace smoking when you experience cravings. You could exercise, visit with a member of your support team, chew gum, eat a healthy snack, and do something to help someone else. Make your own set of choices to replace smoking in your life.

You don't just wake up with a cigarette in your mouth. You make choices that place that cigarette in your mouth and you can use this same power of choice to choose to not smoke. Remember you do have a choice. Will you choose to continue smoking or will you choose to quit smoking today?

Chapter 3- When People Around You Won't Quit

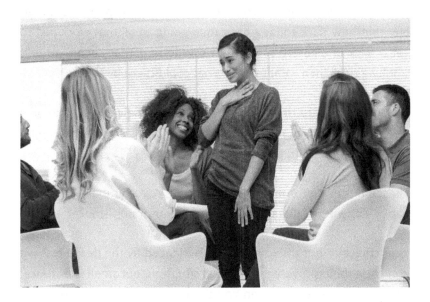

Research has shown that you will improve your success of quitting smoking if you have support or help. Actually your chances of success are up to eight times greater if you work with a support team or program instead of trying to quit smoking by yourself. You do not have to be involved in a formal support program to get the help that you need. You can reach out to family, friends or your physician for this support. You may want to have several different types of support. The more support you have the better your chance of success will be in quitting smoking.

Support is a necessary part of quitting smoking. To obtain support should probably be the first step you make if you really are serious about your desire to quit smoking. Having a support system will provide the needed psychological support. It just could be that this support is all that you need to keep you on the path to quit smoking and to keep your motivation moving along.

Having a good support team will help you when it gets hard to stay on track to successfully stop smoking. It is important to have a support team you trust and that will be available to you.

Complimenting other smoking cessation products with a support program will provide even better results than using the products alone. Remember you may need to select more than one product or source to help you accomplish your goal to quit smoking.

Your support team can even include someone else who is trying to stop smoking at the same time. Yes a quit smoking buddy can replace some of your old smoking buddies providing just the right motivation for you to succeed. This individual can relate to you on the same level regarding what you are experiencing during the time of trying to stop smoking. You can actually be a moral support for each other.

It would probably be good to schedule some routine visits with your quit smoking buddy, this will assure you stay in contact with each other. Make it a social event that can provide additional moral support as you continue to try to stop smoking.

It is very important to have support when you are trying to stop smoking. Identify your quit buddy today or other quit smoking support team and decide to stop smoking today.

One good reason to stop smoking is to stop the hurt that it causes. Yes your decision to quit smoking can stop the hurt to you and others. What better reason could there be to make your decision today.

First you must recognize that smoking is an addiction that causes multiple health issues. Tobacco products contain nicotine, which is an addictive drug. The addictive nature of nicotine can make it very difficult to quit smoking. It has been stated that Nicotine is stronger than many other drugs that some individuals would never consider taking. Often people measure the harmfulness of a product by the number of deaths it causes. So let's take a look this, over 400,000 deaths occur in the United States each year as a result of a smoking related disease. It is a known fact that smoking significantly increases your risk for lung cancer and other types of cancer. It is a reality smoking is not healthy for you. The many effects of smoking are astounding?

When you smoke you are hurting yourself. There is no question at all about this. The question would be what you are going to do about it.

You're Hurting Others

Yes, smoking does hurt others besides you. It can affect your family and others who breathe the smoke created by your cigarettes; this is known as second hand smoke. Second hand smoke is very dangerous and you should consider carefully the harm you are causing to others when you smoke. Sadly to say most of the time second hand smoke is affecting those you truly care about the most your family, children and friends.

Secondhand smoke is responsible for about 300,000 cases of bronchitis and pneumonia in children under the age of 18 months of ages each ear. Secondhand smoke from a parent smoking increases the child's risk for middle ear conditions and creates

Allison McPhee
problems with asthmatic conditions including coughing and wheezing.

In homes where both parents smoke a teenager has twice the risk of smoking than homes where both parents are nonsmokers. Even in homes with only one parent smoking the teenager is more likely to start smoking.

Smoking during pregnancy increases the risk for low birth weights which will affect the health of the infant. If all pregnant women stopped smoking during their pregnancy there would be 4000 less babies to die each year.

If you continue to smoke you are hurting yourself and others.

CHAPTER 4- HOW TO USE A QUIT SMOKING TIMELINE

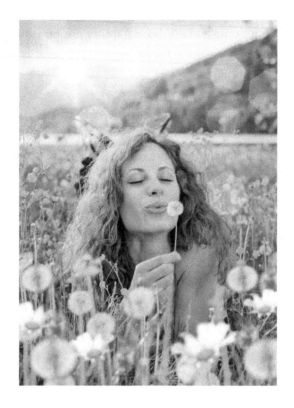

The first step to quit smoking is preparation. In life we have to prepare for most things. We prepare our meals, we prepare to retire for the evening, we prepare for school; we prepare to make a great presentation. So it should not be surprising that when you decide to quit smoking some preparation is needed.

Proper preparation assures for the best change to be successful and well prevent and lessen the problems we may encounter. Preparation to quit smoking will assure your success to stop smoking for your lifetime. Many who fail in their attempt to quit smoking have done so due to lack of preparation. It is estimated that the average smoker has made 6 to 8 attempts to quit before successfully quitting.

Allison McPhee

The first step in preparation is to set a goal. Establish a date you want to stop smoking and improve your health. Do not rush through the preparation steps. It is important to have a good plan to assure you are successful at your attempt to quit smoking. The following points should assist in your preparation.

Take a good look at any previous attempts you have made to quit smoking. When were you most successful? What helped you the most: What didn't work?

Plan for at least 3 months to establish your new behaviors such as exercise, diet and quit smoking. To establish a new habit or lifestyle it is known to take at least 3 months of performing the new behavior or lifestyle routinely to get it established. Do not tack too much at a time. Only try one or two new habits at a time. Doing more will create frustration and actually increase your cravings for tobacco. Do not set yourself up to fail.

- Develop a plan that will provide for 6 or more things to assist with relaxation, handle stress, and keep your hands busy.

- It is best to develop the new habits and then tackle the smoking habit.

- Get a good book about making changes; quit smoking, lifestyle changes etc. to provide assistance along your path to quit smoking.

- You might want to consider the use of nicotine replacement therapy if you are truly addicted to nicotine.

- You may want to consider contacting your doctor regarding the use of medications to assist you with quitting smoking.

- Plan a special way to end your tobacco habit and then stick with you plan

The Quit Smoking Timeline

The landmarks along the pathway to quit smoking are not always the expected ones. There is variation to the quit smoking timeline from person to person. Although the step by step pathway and emotions you encounter may be similar.

The greatest determining factor in how you as an individual handle the process of quitting smoking will be directly related to how Nicotine has affected your brain and body. For an average smoker it takes about 3-4 days for the nicotine to leave your body completely. You may experience withdrawal symptoms that can occur in regular intervals every day.

The first day you may experience difficulty focusing and have unusual feelings. It is important at this landmark to be happy you are doing something for yourself that is good. The next day you may experience restlessness and perhaps develop a strong urge of some kind. It is important to refrain from following these strange but strong urges. This is normal as the nicotine is being removed from your body and chemical changes occur as a result.

By the third day your body will be screaming, you will not have an appetite or taste for food. This is probably one of the most difficult days on the quit smoking timeline. This is the day you must be in full control of yourself. Remember it is important to eat even though you do not have an appetite.

The fourth day you may develop a cough or constipation which are common symptoms. It is time to hang in there, make it through this day and you will awaken to new possibilities.

Now that you made it past day four you will find the quit smoking timeline is a much better approach. At this time you will regain your appetite and your life will seem much more controlled.

Your effort will start to show evidence of return around day 5, It is of utmost importance to maintain consistency throughout the timeline and to be strong not following the various urges you may experience along the way.

You may feel very hungry at times and this may take up to a few months to come back to normal. There are some suggestions in regards to maintain proper dietary intake.

It is important to understand the quit smoking timeline is not the same for everyone. Understanding the timeline and the duration of some of the elements along the timeline may vary

CHAPTER 5- EASY STEPS TO QUIT SMOKING

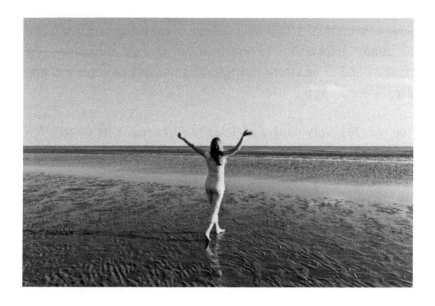

1.Set a Deadline

I underline the term real life quitters as contrary to individuals quitting in the virtual world of the Net individuals who seek out and take part in sites and from time to time spend excessive amounts of time reading and designing how they are going to quit prior to taking the plunge. Some individuals state they were reading for hours or weeks prior to finally trying to quit.

The best individuals to talk to when it concerns stopping smoking are those who have successfully stayed away from smokes for a significant time period. These are individuals who have shown that their strategy in quitting was executable, considering they've quit and are still smoke-free. Speak to everybody you know who's off of nicotine for a year or more and determine how they at the start quit smoking. You'll be astonished at the consistency of the reply you get if you execute that small survey.

Allison McPhee

Individuals are going to pretty much fall under one of the 3 classes of stories. They are:

Individuals, who woke up one day and were all of a sudden, sick and tired of smoking. They pitched them that day and never looked backward.

Individuals who got ill. Not smoking sick, meaning some sort of catastrophic smoking caused sickness. Individuals who got a cold or flu and feel wretched. They feel too sick to smoke, they might feel too ill to eat. They're down with the infection for 2 or 3 days, begin to get better and then recognize that they've a couple of days down without smoking and choose to try to keep it going. Once again, they never look backward and have stuck to their fresh dedication.

Individuals who leave a physician's office and have been given an ultimatum. Stop smoking or kick the bucket - it's your choice. These are individuals for whom some kind of issue has been identified by their physicians, who lay down out in no uncertain terms, that the individuals life is today at risk if they don't stop smoking.

All of these accounts share one matter in common - the strategy that individuals utilize to quit. They merely stop smoking one day. The grounds they quit deviated, but the strategy they utilized was essentially the same. If you have a look at each of the 3 scenarios you'll likewise see that none of them lend themselves to long-run planning - they're spur of the moment determinations provoked by some external condition.

I truly do encourage all individuals to accomplish this survey, speaking to long-run ex-smokers in their real life, individuals who they knew when they were smokers, who they knew when they stopped and who they yet know as ex-smokers. The more individuals do this the more visible it will become how individuals quit smoking and how individuals stay off of smoking. Once again, inhabit stop smoking by merely quitting smoking and individuals stay off of smoking by merely knowing that to stay smoke-free, they must - not pick up another cigarette!

2. Don't Rush Things

Dealing with giving up smoking is no exception. Along with don't pick up another smoke, take each day as it comes is the key strategy which provides the smoker the forte to successfully step down smoking and stay free from the mighty grip of nicotine dependency.

When first stopping, the construct of take each day as it comes is distinctly superior to the smoker believing that he will never smoke again for the remainder of his life. For once the smoker is first ceasing smoking; he doesn't understand whether or not he wishes to go the remainder of his life without smoking. Most of the time, the smoker fancies life as a non-smoker as more nerve-racking, dreadful, and less fun.

It isn't till he stops smoking that he recognizes his prior thoughts of what life is like as a non-smoker were incorrect. Once he stops he recognizes that there's life after smoking. It's a fresher, less agitated, fuller and, most significant, healthier life. Now the thought about returning to smoking gets to be a detestable concept. Even though the fears have lifted, the take-each-day-as-it-comes strategy ought to still be maintained.

Today, as an ex-smoker, he all the same has bad moments every now and again. Occasionally due to tension at home or work, or unpleasant social situations, or to another indefinable trip situation, the want for a cigarette rises. All he needs to do is state to himself, I won't smoke for the remainder of today; tomorrow I'll fret about tomorrow.

The impulse will be over in moments, and the following day he likely won't even consider a cigarette. However take each day as it comes shouldn't only be applied when an impulse is present. It ought to be practiced every day. Occasionally an ex-smoker believes it's no longer crucial to think in these ways.

He goes along with the idea he won't smoke again for the remainder of his life. Presuming he's correct, when does he pat himself on the back for accomplishing his goal? When he's resting on his deathbed he may enthusiastically exclaim, "I never picked up another smoke." What a grand time for positive reward.

Daily the ex-smoker ought to awaken thinking that he isn't going to smoke that day. And nightly before he turns in he ought to compliment himself for sticking with his goal as pride is crucial in remaining free from cigarettes.

Not only is it crucial, but it's well deserved. For anybody who's quit smoking has broken free from a really mighty addiction. For the first time in a long time, he's gained command over his life, instead of being commanded by his cigarette. For this, he ought to be proud.

So this evening, when you turn in, pat yourself on the back and state, "additional day without smoking, I feel grand." And tomorrow once you awaken, state, "I'm going to go for another day. Tomorrow I'll consider tomorrow." To successfully remain free from smoking, take each day as it comes and - never pick up another smoke!

The symptoms of low blood glucose are essentially the same symptoms as not getting enough oxygen, similar to responses experienced at high altitudes. The reason being the poor supply of sugar and/or oxygen means the brain is receiving an incomplete fuel. If you've plenty of one and not plenty of the other, your brain can't operate at any sort of optimum level. Once you stop smoking, oxygen levels are frequently better than they've been in a long time, but with a modified supply of sugar it can't decently fuel your brain.

It isn't that cigarettes place sugar into your blood stream; it's more of a drug interaction of the stimulation effect of nicotine that bears upon the blood glucose levels. Cigarettes drive the body to give up its own stores of sugar and fat by a type of drug interaction. That's how it fundamentally operates as an appetite suppressant, impacting the satiation centers of your hypothalamus. As for the sugar levels, nicotine as a matter of fact works a lot more efficiently than food.

If you utilization food to raise blood glucose levels, it literally calls for up to twenty minutes from the time you chew and swallow the food before it's discharged to the blood, and thus the brain, for its sought after effect of fueling your brain. Cigarettes, by going through a drug interaction get the body to give up its own stores of sugar, but not in twenty minutes but commonly in a matter of moments. In a way, your body hasn't had to give up sugar from food in years; you've done it by utilizing nicotine's drug effect!

This is how come many individuals truly gorge themselves on food upon quitting. They begin to go through a drop in blood glucose and instinctively get hold of something sweet. Upon finishing up the food, they still feel symptoms. Naturally they do, it takes them a moment or two to eat, but the blood glucose isn't hiked up for another eighteen minutes. As they're not feeling instantly better, they consume a bit more. They carry on eating increasingly more food, moment after moment till they at last begin to feel better.

Once again if they're waiting for the blood glucose to go up we're talking of twenty minutes after the 1st swallow. Individuals may eat a lot of food in twenty minutes. But they start to trust that this was the amount required before feeling better. This may be replicated many times throughout the day therefore causing many calories being ingested and inducing weight gain to become a real risk.

Once you suddenly stop smoking, the body is in sort of a state of loss, not willful how to work normally as it hasn't worked normally in such a while. Commonly by the 3rd day, however, your body will readapt and relinquish sugar as it's required. Without consuming any more your body will simply figure out how to govern blood glucose more efficiently.

You might find however that you do have to alter dietary patterns to one that's more regular for you. Regular isn't what it was as a smoker, but more what it was prior to you taking up smoking with aging injected. A few individuals go till evening without eating while they're smokers. If they attempt the same procedure as ex-smokers they'll have side effects of low blood glucose.

It isn't that there has something awry with them now; they were abnormal previously for all pragmatic purposes. This doesn't mean they ought to consume more food, but it might mean they have to redistribute the food consumed to a more disperse pattern so they're getting blood glucose doses throughout the day as nature truly had always intended.

To downplay a few of the true low blood glucose effects of the first few days it truly may help to continue drinking juice throughout the day. After the 4th day however, this ought to no longer be essential as your body ought to be able to give up sugar stores if your diet is normalized.

If you're having issues that are indicative of blood glucose issues beyond day 3, it wouldn't hurt speaking to your physician and perchance acquiring some needed counseling. In order to let your body preserve permanent control over the sum of glucose (sugar) in your brain ... don't pick up another cigarette!

4.Get and Stay Motivated

To state that these individuals had no prior motive or desire to stop smoking would likely not be true. I surmise most smokers have a little level of motivation to stop, but motivation without an understanding of nicotine addiction and its treatment isn't adequate to succeed. That's why most seminars attempt to cram in information as fast as possible.

The crucial things to understand are why individuals smoke, why they ought to stop, how to stop, and how to remain free. All 4 of these areas are essential points of understanding for an individual pondering quitting. Without a firm grasp of each element, the smoker will be disabled in his or her effort to stop.

Understanding why he or she smokes helps the smoker discover that all the magic qualities affiliated with smoking were based on fallacies and feelings. While most smokers believe they smoke because they wish to, the true reason they smoke is because they have to. They're addicted to nicotine and their bodies are requiring that they smoke. They're drug addicts, plain and simple, and realizing this premise is the essential opening move.

Allison McPhee

As with any other addiction or 12-step curriculum, the assumption of being powerless over the drug is the beginning step in recovery. You must realize that while you thought smoking was keeping you calm, it was really increasing your stress levels, or more precisely, your responses to tension. While you believe smoking makes you energetic, in point of fact, it's robbing you of endurance and energy. While smokers frequently feel that smoking allows you to have fun and lead more socially active life-styles, it's really impairing and restricting your power to enlist in many activities and to formulate new relationships.

As contrary to enhancing your power to be vivacious and active members of society, it's in fact inducing you to resort to a lot of asocial behaviors. It led you to smoke in position of human contact, frequently leaving assemblies or declining to attend functions where smoking is no longer permitted. Why an individual ought to quit smoking is likely the least surprising sort of info, as many smokers already understand that smoking is bad for them.

The issue is that most individuals don't realize how bad it is. Many are overpowered when they amply recognize the true magnitude of the perils of smoking. The realization that stopping smoking is in point of fact a battle for survival is often of predominant importance in long-run success. This info is often vital for dealing with the occasional thoughts that are still sparked off by conditions and situations faced throughout the ex-smoker's life.

How to stop - now this is a shock to most: individuals initially quit because they begin to realize smoking is killing them. They then find out that the huge majority of these individuals quit cold turkey. How to remain off, "don't let a err put you back to smoking." That makes as much feel as stating to a recovering alcoholic "don't let a drink put you back to drinking," or a heroin junky being given the message "don't let a little shot put you back to using." The message has to be stronger than that. Not, "don't let a err put you back to using," the message ought to be - do not err!

There has no such thing as an error, or a chance event, or a slip, or a puff, or merely one - they're all terms that are really defining a backsliding! This point is more than any other is what is going to make quitting last. Blanking out this concept, or worse, never acknowledging it all but assures failure.

I've seen the mightiness of education work 1000s of times in helping decently prepare smokers to stop. Again, that issue is more than merely instructing the physical perils of smoking. It means the smoker develops a full grasp of the physical, mental, social, economic, and aesthetic significances of smoking. I've likewise witnessed personal understanding germinate into a mighty tool utilized by 1000s of ex-smokers in keeping up their resolve to stay away from smokes too. They'll carry on maintaining their resolve so long as they go on to appreciate why they quit in the first place, and keeping those reasons in the forefront of their awareness.

May we motivate a smoker to wish to quit? I think many smokers who have smoked cigarettes for any appreciable time period are already motivated. While perhaps not all smokers as a whole, it's likely that any smoker who turns up at a quit smoking clinic on his or her own accord, or who's typed the words "quit smoking" into a Net search engine, has some initial concern and wants more info on how to quit.

So essentially, the answer to whether or not an individual may be motivated to want to quit is "yes." As a matter of fact most smokers already have some motive in place. Understand that to quit smoking and remain off cigarettes and save your life... never pick up another smoke.

Does Hypnosis Help?

An effective hypnosis session to quit smoking can appear to be complicated. Hypnosis encourages behavior change process affection multiple areas of your life. The good thing is you do not have to trouble yourself with getting it together. It will be done for you. The only thing you need to do is use it to improve yourself. You can quit smoking with hypnosis guiding the way.

You are the one with the information regarding your smoking habit. You know very well what creates the strongest craving to smoke for yourself. You also understand the areas of your life that present struggles for you on a daily basis where control is needed.

A well planned hypnosis program will target your specific cravings directly. It will dissolve the emotional triggers making them ineffective. If you have battled with a smoking habit for a lengthy time, you are probably finding it hard to even think of how you would feel without a craving to smoke.

.You can also utilize hypnosis to introduce new cravings for health things, such as drinking water, working out, or simply getting a healthy intake of fresh air. Create a relaxing atmosphere around yourself. Do you have things that need to be done? You can now use the time you previously spent smoking getting things that you want or need done with some time to spare.

Take inventory of your time when smoking:

• How many cigarettes did you smoke per day?

• How many minutes per cigarette?

• How much time spent in a day smoking?

• How much time spent in a week smoking?

Surprising, isn't it? You are probably saying to yourself about now, no wonder I didn't have enough time to get things completed. You were actually robbing yourself of valuable time on a daily basis. After you quit smoking, think of how much more time you will have to simply enjoy living.

Do you experience stress on a daily basis. Without smoking what are you going to do to find relief? Don't worry at all; you can use hypnosis to relieve your stress also. Interesting, don't you agree?

How about your confidence, could it use a boost? Let's try hypnosis to give just the lift that is needed for your confidence. First build confidence and faith in yourself that you can quit smoking this time once and for all. The best part is you can feel absolutely wonderful at the same time. This is probably not your first attempt to quit smoking. Perhaps your previous failures to quit smoking have created just a hint of doubt that this time will end just like all the other times. Well guess what, you can use a little hypnosis to remove that doubt also.

You have probably heart that when you stop smoking watch out for the weight gain, you can also use hypnosis to handle your eating habits. Using hypnosis you can make sure you eating habits stay in control during the time you quit smoking. There is more to the quit smoking process than just simply refraining from smoking and hypnosis can address all of these issues. This should build your confidence of a successful personal quit smoking campaign.

With this well planned hypnosis approach to quit smoking, this time, you will be successful and enter into your own no smoking world. A sound pretty good, doesn't it?

CHAPTER 6 - THE SOCIAL BENEFITS OF NOT SMOKING

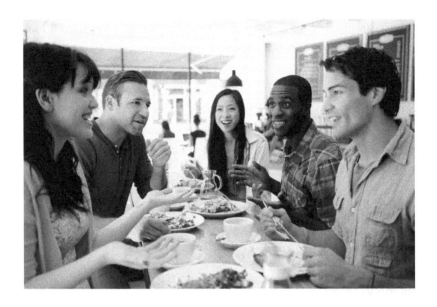

In addition to the many personal benefits to quit smoking, there are also benefits on a social level as well. These social reasons should also be carefully considered in your decision to not smoke.

Social Acceptance

Smoking is not as socially accepted today as it was in past years. Truth is even employers today would rather hire a nonsmoker. Many work environments do not allow for smoking at all or have a very restricted policy regarding smoking. One of the main reasons for this is that there is evidence that employees who smoke increase the cost to the employer by use of sick days more frequently and the effect on the cost of health insurance. Smoking in a facility also increases the cost of maintenance and cleaning to keep odors at an acceptable level.

Locating rental property can also be problematic as many landlords due to maintenance and insurance cost may elect to not rent to smokers. Others may request you not smoke in their homes or vehicles. Most public places today are mostly smoke-free. Entire communities and regions are becoming smoke free in all public areas. Simply finding a place to smoke outside of your own home can be problematic today. That should be an added incentive to quit smoking.

Smoking can limit your opportunities to seek companionship or even marriage, to only smokers which is about 25 percent of the population. Open your playing field by choosing to stop smoking today.

It is really much easier to quit smoking than try to change or adapt the circumstances, things and people around you to accept smoking.

Health of Others

Your smoking will affect the health of those near you. Secondhand smoke exposure is responsible for many deaths from lung cancer and heart disease. Prevent second hand smoke for those around you by quitting smoking now.

Setting an Example for Others

It is your responsibility to set a good example for the children around you. The best way to do this is quit smoking. Most smokers do not want their children or children they are around to start smoking. You can help prevent this by setting an example and stop smoking yourself. Be a good role model for children and don't let them think it is okay to smoke.

Help Is Available

Many ex-smokers are enjoying improved life without smoking each day. You can enjoy the benefits of not smoking by making the decision to stop smoking today. There is no better time to quit smoking than today and start discovering real happiness.

CHAPTER 7- PROCRASTINATION BEATS YOUR PLANS OF STOPPING TO SMOKE

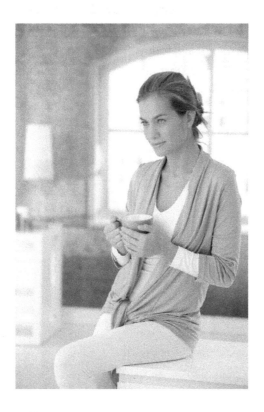

Putting things off, better known as procrastination, is a problem for most people. It may be taking care of the paper work, taking the trash out or perhaps it has even been to quit smoking. Procrastination is a real problem and prevents you from obtaining some very worthwhile goals.

When people put off doing something they know they need to do it leaves them with regrets later. Don't you think it is time to start living life with no regrets? Perhaps you have made the statement "I'm not ready to quit right now, maybe tomorrow" Why wait any longer? You know you need to quit smoking. Just do it.

There is a cost associated with putting things off. Don't pay your bills on time and you will have delinquent charges added on or risk your good credit. Putting off your decision to quit smoking also has a cost. The cost for this could be quite heavy; it could be you pay with your life! It will also continue to cost you the amount you pay for your smoking habit on a daily basis. Start saving now and quit smoking. There are various reasons to procrastinate on things including your decision to stop smoking including the following:

• Fear of failure

• The unknown

• No motivation

• Need for information

• Too many choices

• Failure to make a decision

• Not knowing where to begin

• Not enough time

• Too much work

The reasons are actually just excuses for procrastinating, putting off for later something that should be done now. What would be your excuse today for not quitting smoking? The cure for procrastination is rather simple. Just do it. Now. Today. Do not wait any longer. Make that decision. Just do it. There will never be that perfect time or that perfect product to assist you in quitting smoking. So go on get to it. Make your decision now don't put it off any longer. Live your life without regrets and smoke free.

It can be done one day at a time.

If someone asked you to smoke 8.000 cigarettes today, you would probably tell them it is impossible to do so. But if they told you to smoke 8 cigarettes today that would be a different story. Look at quitting smoking the same way. Decide not to smoke today and then tomorrow decide not to smoke another day. Take one day at a time. The first step to not procrastinating is doing it today. Now go get to it. Stop smoking today.

Why Do You Want to Stop?

Okay it is time to relax. Just get yourself settled in some wonderful assistance on your path to quit smoking.

The reasons you desire to quit smoking are very private and are specifically yours. You own them. They will be the reason you are successful in your attempt to quit smoking this time. That's right your desire to quit smoking does not belong to anyone else at all.

It will be you who makes this journey to a smoke free life. You may have a support team but that is what they will be a support team. This is your journey. This will be your accomplishment.

The path to quit smoking is different for each individual and your case is no exception. It is important to include in your plan the things that will work for you. Oh, you are not sure what will work! Don't worry. You can add to and take away from your plan as you go. The important thing is you have a plan. This is your journey but that does not mean you cannot have help along the way, look at what is available and make your best choice.

There is a goal and that is to quit smoking, enjoy life abundantly in a wealthier, happier, and healthier way. Ready. Let's get started.

There is no magic to this journey that is correct there is no magic carpet or even a magic pill. It will be your desire that brings you to victory lane. It is highly suggested you write down your desires for quitting smoking. As with most road trips they can get long and hard sometimes and you may need to pull out your desire list and review it to assure you are still on the right path.

For whatever reasons you have a smoking habit and you have decided to quit smoking. Do not dwell upon the reasons you started smoking but instead focus on your desires to quit smoking. This will assure your success. You may even find new desires to quit smoking along the path. That is perfectly fine but do make sure you add them to your desire list.

I know you are aware of the dangers in smoking and more than likely the risks associated with these dangers are probably even on your desire list. We will not dwell upon those known dangers. We want to move on from them not stay with them. Any way scare tactics usually do not work and if they do they can have a short life before any time at all the old habits settles right back in. But with your desire list you are always looking ahead reaching for that goal.

You will discover along the path that your desire list will take away the excuses and eventually even the urge to have that next cigarette. Take your desires and run with them. Yes the desire list is the first step but any journey is one step at a time.

CHAPTER 8- WHAT TO EXPECT WHEN YOU'VE STOPPED

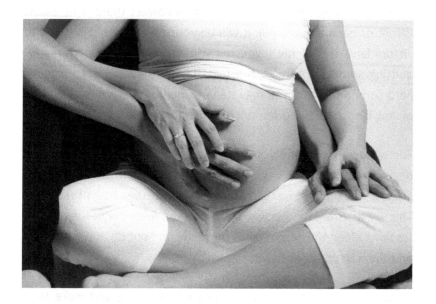

The Cold Turkey

To quit cold turkey is an illusion out of my reach for many smoking two packs of cigarettes a day. It may be the most well-known method to quit smoking and the oldest. If some people try to quit smoking cold turkey, they would be climbing the walls without a plan to act on doing the cold turkey idea. There are alternatives to the cold turkey plan and you may need to try several different plans until you find the right one for you to be successful.

Quit smoking products can be very useful. These products often ease the cravings from nicotine withdrawal. A nicotine patch or gum can be beneficial in an individual's plan of not smoking. If you end up having a few cigarette after you quit just start once again. There is an old saying, if at first you do not succeed just try again. Be creative in ways to stop smoking. The true secret is to not give up. Your final success with be worth the pan and challenges.

A lot of stop smoking products on the market today contain nicotine. There are more stop smoking products coming into the markets that do not contain nicotine. Physicians have many medications available that can be used in a quit smoking program. Bupropion, Chantix, and Fluoxetine are just a few medications available without nicotine. Discuss this with you physician, he will know what is best for our situation.

In the first 48 hours of a stop smoking program you may feel fatigues, irritated or even like a cold is coming on. After the first 48 hours of torture you will feel these feeling began to lessen. Understanding this will be beneficial as you continue our journey to a smoke free life. This knowledge can make the difference between your success and failure.

Need more initiative to quit smoking, consider the financial impact this will have for you as an individual. Let's consider some benefits of not smoking. For an individual smoking two packs of cigarettes a day would equate to about 2,600 dollars. Now that is a big incentive! Let's look at some other incentives to quit smoking:

• Having to go outside in the winter to smoke

• New taxes on cigarettes

• New anti-smoking laws

It is worth it to seriously consider a plan to quit smoking. You will discover many benefits to not smoking including increased wealth and health.

It is always the right time to quit smoking. The sooner you decide to stop smoking and remove the continual punishment smoking puts upon your body the sooner you can be on the road to recovery from years of abuse. Our bodies are magnificently made and can renew itself once harmful substances are removed. As soon as you stop smoking your body will experience improvements immediately as it will not have to try to accommodate the effects of smoking. Your body will have more to overcome the longer you have smoked, but it will return to a healthier state.

Within 20 minutes of your last cigarette your body will begin to return to normal. A natural level of stabilization for both you blood pressure and your pulse rate will be obtained. With improvement of circulation the temperature of your extremities will increase to a normal level as recovery of the arteries is obtained. The carbon monoxide level in your blood drops after about 8 hours from your last cigarette due to increased oxygen in your blood. Brain and muscle function are both affected by the reduction in the amount of oxygen available to inadequate levels.

"Smokers breath" will decrease or be eliminated after you quit smoking. You can see the long term benefits within 24 hours of ceasing to smoke

To quit smoking today will start your lung capacity will begin to show signs of improvement with an average improvement of 30% in just 3 short months.

1 month to 9 months after you have quit smoking you will experience many health improvements including the following

• Less coughing

Allison McPhee

- Less wheezing

- Less sinus congestion

- Less shortness of breath

- Increased energy

- Reduction in chance of infection, especially in the sinuses

- Improved lung function

- A reduction in the risk of coronary heart disease will be obtained after you have quit smoking for one year.

After 5 years of being smoke-free the average smoker who smoked one pack of cigarettes a day will have decreased their lung cancer death rate by almost a half. The risk of developing cancer of the mouth, throat or esophagus will now be half that of a smoker. Remaining smoke-free for 5 to 15 years result in the reduction of your risk for stroke compared to that of a smoker. Approximately 10 years being smoke free your lung cancer death rate will be the same as that of a non-smoker. Healthy cells gradually replace pre-cancerous cells in the body; therefore, reducing the risk of cancer of various types by a considerable percentage. After refraining from smoking 15 years your risk of heart disease is eliminated to that of the nonsmoker These are only a few of the physical improvements that you will experience when you quit smoking. You should recognize the fact that the longer you smoked the longer it will take for your body to reduce the risk smoking as placed upon your body. It is never too late to quit smoking and starting gaining the health benefits you will have.

Books are filled with the reason to quit smoking and the excuses why people don't quit. But if you are pregnant you have an added reason to quit smoking today. Even if you are just planning to have a baby and are smoking consider stopping at this time. The most important reason of all to do so is not for your health but for the health of your unborn child.

Smoking and Birth Weight

Every time you smoke a cigarette and you are pregnant you unborn baby smokes, too. Babies of women who smoke usually will have a lower birth weight than those babies whose mothers are nonsmokers. If you smoke more than a pack of cigarettes a day while pregnant your baby's birth weight will even be lower. A low birth weight puts babies at additional risk. The effects are lingering, in fact a low birth baby from the mother smoking at age 7 will still be smaller than the average child at the same age.

Smoking and Infant Mortality

Infant mortality statistics indicate the risk of infant death at birth or by miscarriage is 50% higher if the mother smokes. Babies of smokers have a 2 ½ times higher risk of dying from sudden infant death syndrome. On the bright side, if you stop smoking by the fourth month of pregnancy these risks will be reduced significantly.

Smoking and Your Health

The health of the mother is also important. Parenting roles are very demanding and require the best health possible. Individuals who smoke put their lives at risk for serious conditions that can be life threatening. A mother needs to be there for her children and if she has put her health at risk by smoking this may not be possible. Lung cancer takes the life of 30,000 women a year. It is important for mothers to stop smoking now so they can remove the risk that could prevent them from being there for their children

Your Family's Health

Passive smoke is dangerous and if you are smoking you are putting your family's health at risk. This is especially true for children.

The Benefits of Quitting

Your unborn child will have the chance to be born healthy if you make the decision to quit smoking. This is not only true for mothers but is also true for fathers.

With children becoming a part of the family make it a family project to provide a smoke free home for your children.

Chapter 9 - Help Yourself Help Others

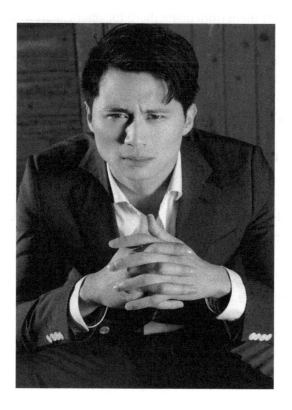

• Forgive Yourself

Do you have guilt or shame for smoking? A lot of people who smoke do feel shame due to the fact they do not control their urge to smoke. Some will even hide the fact that they smoke fearing what others will think of them. Sometimes smokers think they have smoked for so long they should just keep smoking and no try to quit smoking.

Guilt and shame can immobilize an individual. No matter how long someone has smoked they need first to forgive themselves for not quitting sooner. They may come up with a million excuses of why they have not stopped smoking and in their mind this is there way of forgiving themselves. But this is only giving excuses for not stopping to smoke. An excuse denies there is even a problem. Forgives recognizes the problem and then does something about the problem. In order for a smoker to truly forgive them they must move to the next step of deciding to quit smoking.

Forgiveness requires acknowledgement that there is a problem. Yes smoking is a problem. And the smoker desiring to quit but acknowledge that their smoking is a problem. Then they can forgive themselves for the money that has been wasted, perhaps the disobedience if they smoked when their parents did not approve, for the damage the smoking has done to their body. Whatever it is they must forgive themselves and then determine to make a change that is to correct the problem.

Forgiveness allows for a new beginning. When you decide to stop smoking it is the first day for the rest of your life. It is a new beginning. On the other side of quilt by way of forgiveness an individual actually gains control and more freedom. Aren't you ready to be free from your habit of smoking?

It is time to move past smoking and the reasons or excuses of why you even started smoking in the first place. Let forgiveness be a part of today for your past and get on with living life to its' fullest smoke free. You can move past the quilt of yesterday with forgiveness today and quit smoking without delay.

By forgiveness you can look forward with great anticipation and expectation for a wonderful life without regrets. Start the first day of the rest of your life smoke free now today by deciding to quit smoking.

• Gain Weight

Gaining weight may occur with some people when they quit smoking. This has become a concern for meaning when they quit smoking.

It is important to remember that not all people who stop smoking gain weight. The average weight gain is usually between 6 and 8 pounds. Now that should put it in a better perspective for you.

Don't worry, if you are still concerned about gaining even a small amount, let's look at the many ways to prevent a weight gain. No it will not be necessary for you to start a rigid diet at the same time you are trying to quit smoking. There are some very simple tips to assist you and your body to maintain your weight. Give it a try; you may be pleasantly surprised at just how simple it can be.

- First accept who you are and recognize you have made a decision to improve your health by not smoking any longer.

- Exercise moderately such as swimming, jogging, aerobics or playing some type of sport

- Reduce the amount of unhealthy snacks you consume. When you want a snack make a healthy choice of fruit, carrot sticks or other healthy snacks

- Do not drink alcohol or at least limit it to one drink a week

- Maintain a well-balanced diet

- Eat 6 small meals rather than 3 larger meals, this will improve your metabolism throughout the day and you will actually burn more calories

- Increase your water consumption which will help improve your body's metabolism and your body will burn more calories throughout the day. Water will also improve your circulation

- Do not eat past 9pm as the body's metabolism slows down in the evening hours and eating past 9pm will increase the digestion time needed.

Following these rather simple suggestions regarding your dietary habits will help prevent weight gain when you quit smoking. Basically it is changing your eating habits to improve your health and reduce weight gain. Now that you are not smoking you will find the physical activities you can participate in will actually give you more energy.

The health benefits of your decision to quit smoking will far out weight any small weight gain you may experience. Preventing weight gain is much easier than to quit smoking. When you quit smoking other challenges such as weight maintenance will look easy!

- **Bring Back Your Youthful Glory**

Who doesn't want to look good? How we look in important to a lot of aspects of our lives. This is especially important to making good first impressions on others. Smoking does not put you in the best appearance and can affect your first impression on others. Smoking actually ages your complexion.

The effect of smoking on your blood vessels in your skin makes them smaller and prevents a healthy blood flow in this area. Without adequate blood flow your skin is deprived of basic nutrition from collagen, vitamins and minerals. Smoking will actually break down collagen which is the structural protein to maintain elasticity.

With time your skin will begin to dry out appearing old and wrinkled resulting in decline of your complexion. In addition squinting caused from cigarette smoke will actually lead to additional wrinkles. Often you will look as if your smile is replaced with a permanent frown. Stop smoking and wear and smile.

Usually smokers have darkening of their lips which is a typical characteristic of smoking. It is also believed by many experts that dark eye circles are emphasized with smokers. To stop smoking will put the light back into your eyes.

Smoking prevents your skin from healing properly as well. Therefore, injuries and scars take a considerable amount of extra time to heal. Smokers are placed at increased risk for infections and excessive scabbing following surgery or any open wound.

It has been established by research that there is an increased risk of squamous cell carcinoma, a common form of skin cancer, in smokers. In the U.S. annually there are over 1.2 million patients diagnosed with new squamous cell carcinoma.

The skin changes and risk from smoking is actually reversible. After you quit smoking your skin will begin to improve right away. Actually in just a few hours with restoration of circulation the repair process begins and will continue daily. Risk of skin cancer will also be lower after you stop smoking.

Look younger by stopping the damage smoking is doing to your skin now before it is too late. Remember you will start to see the improvements to your complexion within just a few hours of not smoking. Your skin needs the oxygen and nutrients provided by adequate blood flow and smoking limits the blood flow. Make your decision to gain your youthfulness back by not smoking today.

• Help Others to Quit

Do you remember the famous words of parents "Do as I say, not as I do?" I am sure you have heard them and if you are a parent I am very sure you have said them. People always have advice to give away and when it comes to the need to quit smoking it is no different.

Ever notice how advice is given often even when it is not asked for. Everybody has their own opinion and just love to share it with others. Have you ever heard someone tell a smoker, "Just quit it isn't hard"? Often these individuals have never smoked even one cigarette, how would they even know if it is hard to quit smoking or not. One thing for sure giving advice is not hard

If getting advice from others does not help you decide to quit but perhaps if you look for an opportunity to help someone else you can help yourself at the same time. That would be a different approach but let's look how this just might work. You might be surprised to find the benefits awaiting you.

Do you have a teenager and you really do not want them to start smoking. Take this opportunity to help them by allowing them to not only hear you say, "Do as I say", but to also see "do as I do". Be an example for them showing them that smoking is not good for them or you and do this by deciding to quit. Include them as a part of your support team. This example will leave a lasting impression upon them and look you actually received a lifetime of benefits for yourself as well.

If you do not have a teenager, find someone who could benefit from quitting smoking as well and encourage them to quit with you. As you give encouragement and advice to another smoker you will also be encouraging yourself.

You will quickly find that as you give someone else advice on quitting smoking the answers to their challenges will be easy for you to see and then you can apply this to your own effort to quit smoking as well.

The end result will be you have quit smoking and so has another smoker or even better you may have prevented someone else from every having a smoking habit at all. What a lifetime impact helping others can have.

• **Get Back in Shape**

Kicking your smoking habit is probably the hardest thing you will ever do. You will need all the help you can get to successfully quit smoking. Exercise can be helpful with reducing some of your nicotine urges.

In addition to reduce the cravings for nicotine, exercise can also help you to maintain your weight during the time you are trying to stop smoking. Weight gain is a common problem experienced during a smoking cessation program. Perhaps exercising only serves as a distraction from smoking but if so let it be it is still helping. You will obtain some additional benefits from your exercise program in improving your health and weight maintenance.

There are many different types of exercise programs that you can choose from. It should be noted that the type of exercise is not as important as the fact that you are exercising. So choose something that you will enjoy and stick with on a consistent basis.

It will not be necessary for you to buy a membership into a health gym, as you can exercise right where you are and any time you have an urge to have a cigarette.

Perhaps you would like to use a treadmill. If you plan on making a purchase it is important to do some homework first. This will save you both time and money.

First consider ratings for treadmills and then make your selection. Some suggestions for ratings are provided for you here

• Name brand: a recognized brand from an established manufacturer is a safe bet Horsepower: you want least 1.5 continuous hp

• Belt size: it should be at least 17 inches wide and 51 inches long

• Type of deck: a pretreated, no-maintenance, shock-absorbing deck is best

• Safety precautions: look for emergency shut off, handrails, etc.

• Warranty

You can also consider other types of exercise equipment. You might want to talk with someone at a local gym or perhaps your doctor about what type of equipment would be best for you to use.

Perhaps you enjoy biking then by all means use your bike for exercise. If you don't want to use any type of exercise equipment then you can always walk. There is not any better way to exercise than walking and it takes only a comfortable pair of shoes to participate in this type of exercise. Don't let the weather stop you from exercising. You can walk at your local mall or department store inside in any kind of weather.

Put out that cigarette and start exercising your way to a smoke free healthy lifestyle today.

CHAPTER 10 - OTHER TIPS TO HELP YOU STOP SMOKING TODAY

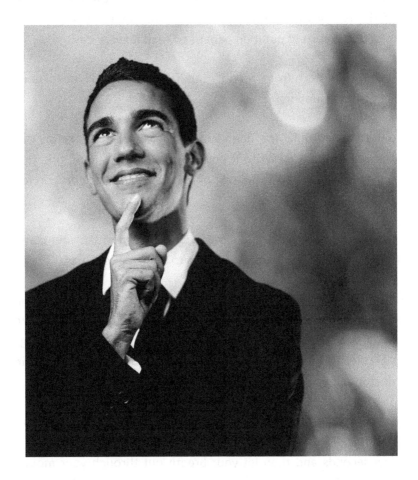

Have you made the decision to quit smoking? Looking for path you can follow with ease and not too complicated? Continue reading for some great quick tips.

- You must believe you can quit and in yourself. Quitting is up to you and you can do it.

- Make a personal plan for quitting smoking. Your own words and your own way. You will follow your own plan better than someone else's.

- Think about the reasons you want to quit. What are the benefits such as living longer, feeling better, perhaps for your family, to save money, rid yourself of smoke odors are just a few of some of the reasons you may have. Now write them down on a list. Yes, that is correct put it on paper and read it every day.

- Ask for support from friends and family. You will need non-judgmental support.

- Set a date to quit. The day you will put your last cigarettes out forever. You got it. Write it down. Perhaps you should title this paper "the first day of the rest of my life". Plan a celebration for this day.

- Make an appointment and discuss with your physician your plans to stop smoking. Add your physician to your support team.

- Start an exercise program. This will prove to help reduce your stress and assist your recovery from the cigarette damage your body has received over the years you have been smoking. Consider this a gift to your body. You should also talk with your doctor about this as well.

- Every day perform deep breathing for 3-5 minutes. Do this by breathing in through your nose slowly, hold your breath a just a few seconds and then let your breath out through your mouth very slowly. You may even want to close your eyes when doing deep breathing.

- Imagine yourself as a non-smoker. Do this during the deep breathing for added benefits. Perhaps you see yourself dramatically tossing your cigarettes over a bridge or see yourself riding a bike in a marathon. Whatever works for you make a visual picture of it and pull it out every now and then to gain energy?

- Start by cutting back on the number of cigarettes you smoke if you just can't stop suddenly. Always work toward your quit date you have established.

- Use the cold turkey method. Some smokers find the only way to quit is to simply stop smoking without trying first to cut back. If cutting back doesn't work for you try going cold turkey?

- Partner with another smoker who also wants to quit. Become quit buddies helping each other along the way to a smoke free life.

- Make a Dentist appointment. Yes, you read that correctly. Make an appointment with your Dentist to have your teeth cleaned. Like that bright smile, keep it that way Stop smoking now.

- Plan a celebration to celebrate different goals you attain on your way. Ideas can be the day you quit, 1 week with no smoking, 1 month, it doesn't matter what the milestones you set are but that you set them and then celebrate. You deserve it.

- Increase your intake of water. Water will help cleanse your body of the nicotine.

- Identify what increases your desire for a cigarette and then avoid it. Make some life style changes that will complement your effort to stop smoking.

- Replace the cigarette you are used to holding with another object. You might consider a pen or straw.

- Write a poem or song about quitting cigarettes and then read it daily. Don't feel real creative use a song of your choice and replace some of the words to accomplish your own quit smoking song. Sing it each day as you shower.

- Get a picture of someone important to you and writ a not that says "I'm will quit smoking for you" tape in on the picture and carry the picture with you. Whenever you have an urge to smoke simply pull the picture out and read the message you have written.

- Start a journal and write it in along your quit smoking path.

ABOUT THE AUTHOR

Allan Doe is a lifestyle manager and a licensed therapist. He handles celebrities and other notable family. His job includes the management of personal net worth with the end goal of making a client look better.

Allan was raised into a family of smokers but he never caught the habit. He attributes his vehement resistance to nicotine to seeing his own father die of lung cancer and his mother suffer several miscarriages.

Today, Allan wants to share his knowledge on smoking and second hand smoke to everyone who wants to listen. This book is one of his many awareness campaign methods.

Lightning Source UK Ltd.
Milton Keynes UK
UKHW02f2110051217

313940UK00019B/516/P